Lyme Cure Treatment

Advances and Prevention of Lyme Disease

By

Archie Finley

Table of Contents

CHAPTER 1

Holistic Approaches to Lyme Disease

Diet and Nutrition

Diet and nutrition play a significant role in supporting overall health and well-being, including in the management of Lyme disease. A holistic approach to Lyme disease encompasses not only the use of conventional treatments but also the incorporation of lifestyle modifications, including dietary considerations. The importance of diet and nutrition in managing Lyme disease and provide an in-depth analysis of various aspects of a holistic approach to nutrition.

1. Anti-Inflammatory Diet: Chronic inflammation is a common feature of Lyme disease, and adopting an anti-inflammatory diet can help mitigate inflammation and support the body's healing processes. The key principles of an anti-inflammatory diet include:

- Emphasizing Whole Foods: Prioritizing whole, unprocessed foods such as fruits, vegetables, whole grains, lean proteins, and healthy fats. These foods are rich in essential nutrients, antioxidants, and fiber, which support immune function and reduce inflammation.

- Omega-3 Fatty Acids: Including sources of omega-3 fatty acids in the diet, such as fatty fish (salmon, sardines), flaxseeds, chia seeds, and walnuts. Omega-3 fatty acids have anti-inflammatory properties and can help balance the immune response.

- Phytonutrients: Consuming a variety of colorful fruits and vegetables, as they contain phytonutrients with potent antioxidant and anti-inflammatory properties. Examples include berries, leafy greens, cruciferous vegetables, and herbs like turmeric and ginger.

- Avoiding Processed Foods: Minimizing or avoiding processed and refined foods, which are often high in added sugars, unhealthy fats, and artificial ingredients that can contribute to inflammation.

2. Gut Health and Immune Support: The gut plays a crucial role in immune function, and maintaining a

healthy gut microbiome can support the immune system's ability to fight infections. Consider the following:

- Probiotic-Rich Foods: Incorporating probiotic-rich foods into the diet, such as yogurt, kefir, sauerkraut, and kimchi. These foods introduce beneficial bacteria into the gut, promoting a healthy balance of microorganisms.

- Prebiotic Foods: Including prebiotic foods that nourish the gut bacteria, such as onions, garlic, leeks, asparagus, bananas, and whole grains. Prebiotics serve as fuel for beneficial gut bacteria, supporting their growth and diversity.

- Fiber-Rich Foods: Consuming an adequate amount of dietary fiber from sources like fruits, vegetables, legumes, and whole grains. Fiber promotes regular bowel movements and helps eliminate toxins from the body.

- Hydration: Staying well-hydrated by drinking an adequate amount of water throughout the day. Proper hydration supports digestion, detoxification, and overall health.

3. Nutrient Support: Optimizing nutrient intake can help support the body's immune system and promote healing. Consider the following:

- Antioxidant-Rich Foods: Including foods high in antioxidants, such as berries, citrus fruits, dark leafy greens, nuts, and seeds. Antioxidants help neutralize free radicals, reducing oxidative stress and supporting the immune system.

- Essential Nutrients: Ensuring adequate intake of essential nutrients like vitamins (particularly vitamin C, vitamin D, and B vitamins), minerals (including zinc and selenium), and omega-3 fatty acids. These nutrients are crucial for immune function, energy production, and tissue repair.

- Adequate Protein: Consuming sufficient protein from sources like lean meats, poultry, fish, eggs, legumes, and plant-based proteins. Protein supports tissue repair, immune function, and overall health.

4. Individualized Approaches: It's important to recognize that each individual with Lyme disease may have unique dietary needs and considerations. Some individuals may have specific food sensitivities or allergies, while others may require modifications based on co-existing conditions or medication interactions. Consulting with a healthcare provider, registered dietitian, or integrative medicine practitioner experienced in Lyme disease can help

tailor a diet plan to individual needs.

5. Avoiding Dietary Triggers: Some individuals with Lyme disease may experience worsened symptoms or increased inflammation in response to certain foods or dietary triggers. These triggers can vary among individuals but may include processed foods, refined sugars, gluten, dairy products, and potential allergens. Keeping a food diary and paying attention to symptom patterns can help identify potential triggers and guide dietary adjustments.

It's important to note that diet and nutrition should complement conventional medical treatments for Lyme disease and not replace them. Always consult with a healthcare provider before making significant changes to your diet or starting any new dietary supplements.

diet and nutrition are essential components of a holistic approach to managing Lyme disease. An anti-inflammatory diet, gut health support, nutrient optimization, and individualized approaches can help support the immune system, reduce inflammation, and promote overall well-being. By incorporating these principles into daily life, individuals with Lyme disease can enhance their healing journey and optimize their health outcomes.

Herbal and Natural Remedies

In addition to conventional treatments, many individuals with Lyme disease explore herbal and natural remedies as part of a holistic approach to their healing journey. These remedies are often used in conjunction with medical interventions and lifestyle modifications to support the immune system, alleviate symptoms, and promote overall well-being. we will delve into the world of herbal and natural remedies commonly considered in the context of Lyme disease.

1. Herbal Remedies:

Herbal remedies have been used for centuries in various traditional systems of medicine for their potential therapeutic properties. While research on herbal remedies specifically for Lyme disease is limited, some herbs have gained attention for their potential immune-boosting, antimicrobial, and anti-inflammatory effects. It's important to note that the use of herbal remedies should be approached with caution, and it is advisable to consult with a healthcare professional or a qualified herbalist before incorporating them into a treatment plan. Here are some commonly mentioned herbs for Lyme disease:

- Japanese Knotweed (Polygonum cuspidatum): Known for its antimicrobial and anti-inflammatory properties, Japanese knotweed is often used as a supportive herb in Lyme disease treatment. It contains resveratrol, a compound with potential antioxidant and immune-modulating effects.

- Cat's Claw (Uncaria tomentosa): Cat's claw is believed to have immune-stimulating and anti-inflammatory properties. It is commonly used in herbal protocols for Lyme disease to support the immune system and alleviate symptoms.

- Andrographis (Andrographis paniculata): Andrographis is traditionally used for its antimicrobial and immune-modulating properties. It has been studied for its potential effectiveness against tick-borne infections and is often included in herbal protocols for Lyme disease.

- Samento (Uncaria tomentosa): Samento is a type of cat's claw extract that is often used in Lyme disease treatment protocols. It is believed to have antimicrobial properties and may support immune function.

- Garlic (Allium sativum): Garlic is well-known for its antimicrobial properties and immune-supportive effects. It is often included in natural treatment approaches for Lyme disease due to its potential

broad-spectrum
antimicrobial activity.

2. Natural Remedies:

In addition to herbal remedies,
several natural remedies are
commonly considered in the
context of Lyme disease. These
remedies may help support the
body's healing processes and
alleviate symptoms. It is
important to note that scientific
research on their effectiveness in
Lyme disease is limited, and
individual responses may vary.
Here are some commonly
mentioned natural remedies for
Lyme disease:

- Essential Oils: Certain
  essential oils, such as

oregano, tea tree, and clove, are believed to possess antimicrobial properties and may be used in topical applications or aromatherapy to address symptoms associated with Lyme disease. However, it is crucial to use essential oils safely, following proper dilution guidelines and consulting with a qualified aromatherapist or healthcare provider.

- Probiotics: Probiotics are beneficial bacteria that can help support a healthy gut microbiome and immune function. While not specific to Lyme disease, maintaining a healthy balance of gut bacteria through probiotic supplementation or probiotic-rich foods may support overall health and immune function.

- Nutritional Supplements: Certain nutritional supplements may be considered to address specific nutrient deficiencies or support immune function. These may include vitamins (such as vitamin C, vitamin D, and B vitamins), minerals (such as zinc and selenium), and other compounds like coenzyme

Q10 and alpha-lipoic acid.
However, it is important to
consult with a healthcare
provider to determine
appropriate dosages and
ensure compatibility with
other treatments or
medications.

3. Individual Considerations:

The use of herbal and natural
remedies should be
individualized and take into
account factors such as the
severity of symptoms, overall
health, potential interactions with
medications, and personal
sensitivities. It is advisable to
work closely with a
knowledgeable healthcare

provider or integrative medicine practitioner experienced in Lyme disease to develop a comprehensive treatment plan that incorporates herbal and natural remedies.

4. Safety and Quality Considerations:

When considering herbal and natural remedies, it is crucial to prioritize safety and quality. Here are some important considerations:

- Quality Control: Ensure that the herbs or natural products are sourced from reputable suppliers who adhere to good manufacturing practices and undergo third-party testing for purity and potency.

- Professional Guidance: Seek guidance from qualified healthcare professionals, such as naturopathic doctors, herbalists, or integrative medicine practitioners who have experience in treating Lyme disease. They can provide personalized recommendations and monitor your progress.

- Potential Interactions: Be aware of potential interactions between herbal remedies and conventional

medications. Some herbs
may interfere with the
efficacy or safety of certain
medications, and it is
important to discuss any
herbal or natural remedies
with your healthcare
provider to avoid potential
adverse effects.

- Allergic Reactions and
  Sensitivities: Individuals
  may have individual
  sensitivities or allergies to
  certain herbs or natural
  remedies. It is essential to
  be aware of any allergic
  reactions or adverse effects
  and discontinue use if
  necessary.

herbal and natural remedies are often considered as part of a holistic approach to Lyme disease. While research on their effectiveness specifically for Lyme disease is limited, some herbs and natural remedies may offer immune-boosting, antimicrobial, or anti-inflammatory properties. However, it is crucial to approach their use with caution, seek professional guidance, and prioritize safety and quality. Integrating herbal and natural remedies into a comprehensive treatment plan, alongside conventional medical interventions and lifestyle modifications, may help support overall well-being and complement the management of Lyme disease.

Lifestyle Changes and Self-Care

In addition to medical treatments and alternative remedies, incorporating lifestyle changes and self-care practices is a vital aspect of a holistic approach to managing Lyme disease. These changes aim to support overall well-being, enhance the body's healing capabilities, and improve the quality of life for individuals with Lyme disease. we will explore various lifestyle changes and self-care practices that can be beneficial in the context of Lyme disease.

1. Rest and Sleep: Adequate rest and quality sleep are essential for healing and supporting the immune system. Lyme disease can often lead to fatigue, insomnia, and disrupted sleep patterns. Prioritizing rest and establishing healthy sleep habits can contribute to overall well-being. Here are some strategies:

- Establish a Routine: Establish a regular sleep schedule by going to bed and waking up at consistent

times each day, even on
weekends.

- Create a Restful
  Environment: Create a calm
  and relaxing sleep
  environment by ensuring a
  comfortable mattress and
  pillows, adjusting room
  temperature, and
  minimizing noise and light
  disturbances.

- Relaxation Techniques:
  Engage in relaxation
  techniques before bedtime,
  such as deep breathing
  exercises, meditation, or
  listening to calming music,
  to promote relaxation and
  better sleep.

- Limit Stimulants: Avoid stimulants like caffeine and electronic devices close to bedtime, as they can interfere with sleep quality.

2. Stress Management: Stress can exacerbate symptoms and impact overall well-being. Developing effective stress management techniques can help individuals with Lyme disease better cope with the challenges they face. Consider the following strategies:

- Mindfulness and Meditation: Engage in mindfulness practices, such

as meditation or deep
breathing exercises, to
cultivate a sense of calm
and reduce stress levels.

- Physical Activity: Engage
in gentle physical activities,
such as walking, yoga, or
tai chi, which can help
reduce stress, improve
mood, and enhance overall
well-being. However, it is
important to tailor physical
activity to individual
abilities and consult with a
healthcare provider.

- Time Management:
Prioritize tasks and
establish realistic goals to
avoid feeling overwhelmed.

Breaking tasks into
manageable steps and
delegating, when necessary,
can help reduce stress
levels.

- Relaxation Techniques:
Explore relaxation
techniques such as
progressive muscle
relaxation, guided imagery,
or aromatherapy to promote
relaxation and reduce
stress.

3. Balanced Nutrition:
Adopting a balanced and
nourishing diet can support
the body's healing
processes, boost immune

function, and promote overall well-being.

4. Gentle Exercise and Movement: Physical activity should be approached with caution, considering individual energy levels and symptom severity. Engaging in gentle exercises and movement can provide numerous benefits, including:

- Increased Circulation: Gentle exercises, such as stretching, walking, or light yoga, can improve blood circulation, which aids in the delivery of nutrients and removal of toxins.

- Improved Mood: Physical activity releases endorphins, which can improve mood and reduce feelings of anxiety or depression.

- Enhanced Energy and Stamina: Regular, gentle exercises can improve overall energy levels and stamina over time. It is important to start slowly and gradually increase activity levels, listening to the body's cues.

5. Environmental Considerations: Creating a supportive and healthy environment can contribute

to overall well-being. Some considerations include:

- Reducing Environmental Toxins: Minimize exposure to environmental toxins, such as pesticides, chemicals, and mold, which can exacerbate symptoms and compromise immune function. This may involve using natural cleaning products, improving indoor air quality, and ensuring proper ventilation.

- Outdoor Safety: Taking precautions when spending time outdoors, such as wearing protective clothing, using insect repellent, and

checking for ticks, can help
reduce the risk of additional
tick bites and potential co-
infections.

- Emotional Support:
Surround yourself with a
supportive network of
family, friends, or support
groups who understand the
challenges of living with
Lyme disease. Seek
emotional support when
needed, as it can greatly
impact mental well-being.

6. Self-Care Practices:
Engaging in self-care
practices is essential for
maintaining overall well-
being and managing the

emotional toll of Lyme disease. Here are some self-care activities to consider:

- Relaxation Techniques: Practice relaxation techniques, such as deep breathing exercises, meditation, or progressive muscle relaxation, to reduce stress and promote a sense of calm.

- Creative Outlets: Engage in creative activities that bring joy and help express emotions, such as painting, writing, playing music, or gardening.

- Mind-Body Techniques: Explore mind-body

practices like yoga, tai chi, or qigong, which integrate physical movement, breathwork, and mindfulness to promote relaxation and overall well-being.

- Pamper Yourself: Treat yourself to activities that promote self-care and relaxation, such as taking baths, practicing aromatherapy, receiving massages, or engaging in hobbies that bring joy and relaxation.

incorporating lifestyle changes and self-care practices is crucial in managing Lyme disease holistically. Prioritizing rest, managing stress, adopting a balanced diet, engaging in gentle exercise, creating a healthy environment, and practicing self-care activities can contribute to overall well-being and enhance the body's healing capabilities. It is important to personalize these strategies to individual needs, listen to the body's cues, and work closely with healthcare professionals experienced in Lyme disease management to ensure the most effective and safe approach.

Complementary Therapies

In addition to conventional medical treatments and lifestyle modifications, many individuals with Lyme disease explore complementary therapies as part of their holistic approach to managing the condition. Complementary therapies are non-conventional treatments that aim to support overall well-being, alleviate symptoms, and promote healing. While the effectiveness of these therapies for Lyme disease may vary among individuals, they can be valuable additions to a comprehensive treatment plan. we will explore some commonly used complementary therapies for Lyme disease.

1. Acupuncture: Acupuncture is a traditional Chinese

medicine practice that
involves inserting thin
needles into specific points
on the body. It is believed
to stimulate energy flow
and restore balance in the
body. Acupuncture has
been used by some
individuals with Lyme
disease to manage pain,
reduce inflammation, and
support overall well-being.
It is important to consult
with a licensed
acupuncturist who is
experienced in working
with individuals with Lyme
disease to ensure safety and
effectiveness.

2. Massage Therapy: Massage therapy involves the manipulation of soft tissues in the body to promote relaxation, relieve muscle tension, and improve circulation. It can be beneficial for individuals with Lyme disease who experience muscle pain, stiffness, and tension. Massage therapy may also help reduce stress and promote a sense of well-being. It is advisable to work with a licensed massage therapist who understands the specific needs and sensitivities of

individuals with Lyme
disease.

3. Chiropractic Care:
Chiropractic care focuses
on the alignment of the
musculoskeletal system,
particularly the spine, to
promote overall health and
well-being. Some
individuals with Lyme
disease may experience
musculoskeletal issues,
such as joint pain or
misalignment, that can be
addressed through
chiropractic adjustments. It
is important to consult with
a qualified chiropractor
who has experience
working with individuals

with Lyme disease to ensure appropriate care and avoid exacerbation of symptoms.

4. Energy Healing: Energy healing practices, such as Reiki, Healing Touch, or Qigong, work with the body's energy fields to promote balance, relaxation, and overall well-being. These therapies are based on the belief that disruptions in energy flow can contribute to physical and emotional imbalances. While scientific evidence regarding the effectiveness of energy healing for Lyme disease is limited, some

individuals find these practices helpful in managing stress, promoting relaxation, and supporting their healing journey.

5. Herbal Medicine: Herbal medicine, also known as botanical medicine, involves the use of plant-based remedies to support healing and alleviate symptoms. Herbal remedies have been used for centuries in various traditional systems of medicine and can be beneficial for individuals with Lyme disease. However, it is important to consult with a qualified

herbalist or healthcare provider experienced in treating Lyme disease to ensure appropriate use and avoid potential interactions with medications.

6. Mind-Body Techniques: Mind-body techniques aim to harness the connection between the mind and the body to promote healing and overall well-being. These techniques include practices such as meditation, mindfulness, guided imagery, and relaxation exercises. Mind-body techniques can help reduce stress, enhance resilience, and improve the

body's response to
treatment. Incorporating
these techniques into daily
life can provide individuals
with Lyme disease with
valuable tools for managing
symptoms and improving
quality of life.

7. Naturopathy: Naturopathy
is a holistic approach to
healthcare that focuses on
supporting the body's
natural healing abilities.
Naturopathic physicians
may incorporate a range of
treatments, including herbal
medicine, nutritional
counseling, lifestyle
modifications, and other
natural therapies, to address

the individual needs of patients with Lyme disease. Working with a qualified naturopathic physician who specializes in Lyme disease can provide personalized guidance and support.

It is important to note that while complementary therapies can be valuable additions to a holistic treatment plan, they should not replace conventional medical care for Lyme disease. It is essential to work closely with healthcare professionals, including Lyme-literate doctors or integrative medicine practitioners, who can provide comprehensive guidance and monitor the progress of treatment.

complementary therapies offer additional options for individuals with Lyme disease to support their healing journey and enhance their overall well-being. Acupuncture, massage therapy, chiropractic care, energy healing, herbal medicine, mind-body techniques, and naturopathy are among the many complementary therapies that individuals may explore. It is important to approach these therapies with an open mind, seek qualified practitioners, and communicate openly with healthcare providers to ensure safe and effective integration into a comprehensive treatment plan.

CHAPTER 2

Cutting-Edge Research and Emerging Treatments

Advances in Lyme Disease Research

Lyme disease research has made significant progress in recent years, leading to a better understanding of the disease and the development of innovative diagnostic techniques and treatment approaches. We will explore some of the cutting-edge research and emerging treatments that are shaping the field of Lyme disease.

1. Improved Diagnostic Methods: One area of advancement in Lyme disease research is the development of improved diagnostic methods. Traditional diagnostic tests for Lyme disease, such as the enzyme-linked immunosorbent assay (ELISA) and Western blot, have limitations in terms of sensitivity and specificity, leading to potential false-negative results. However, researchers have been working on developing

more accurate and reliable diagnostic tools.

One notable advancement is the development of next-generation sequencing (NGS) techniques, which allow for the detection of a broader range of pathogens and provide more comprehensive information about the infection. NGS can identify not only the Borrelia burgdorferi bacteria but also other potential co-infections that may occur alongside Lyme disease. This advancement in diagnostic methods can lead to earlier detection, more accurate diagnosis, and improved treatment outcomes.

2. Vaccine Development:
    Vaccine development has
    been a significant area of
    focus in Lyme disease
    research. In the past, a
    Lyme disease vaccine
    called LYMErix was
    available but was
    withdrawn from the market
    due to low demand and
    concerns over potential side
    effects. However,
    researchers continue to
    explore new vaccine
    candidates.

One promising vaccine candidate
is based on a protein called
OspA, found on the surface of
the Borrelia burgdorferi bacteria.
This vaccine aims to stimulate

the immune system to produce
antibodies against OspA,
preventing the bacteria from
causing an infection. Several
experimental OspA-based
vaccines are currently in
development and undergoing
clinical trials, showing promising
results in terms of safety and
efficacy.

3. Novel Antibiotic Therapies:
   The development of novel
   antibiotic therapies is
   another area of active
   research in Lyme disease.
   While antibiotics are
   currently the mainstay of
   Lyme disease treatment,
   there is ongoing research to
   identify more effective

antibiotics, improve treatment regimens, and address antibiotic resistance.

Researchers are exploring alternative antibiotics, such as those from different classes or combinations of antibiotics, to target persistent or antibiotic-resistant forms of the Borrelia bacteria. Additionally, drug repurposing efforts are underway to identify existing drugs that may have activity against Lyme disease, potentially offering more treatment options.

4. Host-Directed Therapies: Host-directed therapies are a new and promising

approach to treating Lyme disease. These therapies focus on modulating the host's immune response to combat the infection. The goal is to enhance the body's immune defenses against the Borrelia bacteria and reduce the severity of symptoms.

Immunomodulatory drugs, such as those used in autoimmune diseases, are being explored for their potential in Lyme disease treatment. These drugs can help regulate the immune system, reduce inflammation, and enhance the body's ability to fight off the infection. Clinical trials are ongoing to evaluate the safety and efficacy of these host-directed therapies in Lyme disease.

5. Precision Medicine: Advances in genomics and personalized medicine have the potential to revolutionize Lyme disease treatment. Precision medicine aims to tailor medical treatment to individual patients based on their unique genetic makeup, immune response, and other relevant factors. In the context of Lyme disease, precision medicine may help identify individuals who are more susceptible to severe

symptoms, determine the
optimal treatment approach,
and predict treatment
outcomes.

Genetic testing and immune
profiling are being utilized to
identify biomarkers that can
guide treatment decisions and
improve patient outcomes. By
understanding the individual
characteristics and genetic
variations that influence disease
progression and treatment
response, healthcare providers
can offer more personalized and
targeted therapies.

6. Emerging Therapies:
   Several emerging therapies
   are being explored in

preclinical and early clinical stages for the treatment of Lyme disease. These include:

- Photodynamic Therapy: Photodynamic therapy involves the use of light and a photosensitizing agent to destroy pathogens. It shows promise in targeting Borrelia bacteria while minimizing damage to surrounding healthy tissues.

- Immunotherapies: Immunotherapies, such as monoclonal antibodies or immune checkpoint inhibitors, are being investigated to boost the immune system's response against the Borrelia bacteria and enhance the effectiveness of antibiotic treatment.

- Antimicrobial Peptides: Antimicrobial peptides are small molecules with potent antimicrobial properties. Researchers are investigating the use of these peptides to target and kill Borrelia bacteria.

- Microbiome-Based Therapies: The microbiome, the collection of microorganisms in our body, plays a crucial role in our health. Researchers are studying the potential of microbiome-based therapies, such as probiotics or fecal microbiota transplantation, to modulate the immune response and improve treatment outcomes in Lyme disease.

It is important to note that while these advancements in research hold promise for the future, further studies and clinical trials are needed to establish their safety, efficacy, and optimal use in Lyme disease treatment. Close collaboration between researchers, healthcare providers, and patients is essential to translate these cutting-edge research findings into effective and accessible treatments for individuals with Lyme disease.

ongoing research in Lyme disease is paving the way for improved diagnostic methods, the development of new vaccines, novel antibiotic therapies, host-directed therapies, precision medicine approaches, and the exploration of emerging treatment modalities. These advancements offer hope for more accurate diagnosis, effective treatments, and better management of Lyme disease, ultimately improving the quality of life for those affected by this complex condition.

Immunotherapy and Vaccines

Immunotherapy and vaccines are emerging as promising areas of research in the field of Lyme disease. These innovative approaches aim to harness the body's immune system to combat the Borrelia burgdorferi bacteria and prevent or treat Lyme disease. we will explore the cutting-edge research and emerging treatments related to immunotherapy and vaccines.

1. Immunotherapy:
   Immunotherapy refers to the use of therapeutic agents that modulate the immune system to enhance

its response against the Borrelia bacteria. This approach recognizes that the immune system plays a critical role in controlling infections and seeks to bolster its effectiveness. Several immunotherapy strategies are being investigated for Lyme disease:

- Monoclonal Antibodies: Monoclonal antibodies are laboratory-produced antibodies that specifically target and neutralize certain molecules or pathogens. In the context of Lyme disease, researchers are developing monoclonal antibodies that bind to the surface proteins of the Borrelia bacteria, impairing their ability to infect host cells and promoting their clearance by the immune system.

- Immune Checkpoint Inhibitors: Immune checkpoint inhibitors are a class of drugs that help unleash the immune system's ability to recognize and attack cancer cells. Some studies suggest that immune checkpoint inhibitors may also have potential in Lyme disease treatment by boosting the immune response against

the Borrelia bacteria.
However, more research is
needed to evaluate their
safety and efficacy in this
context.

- Cytokine Therapies:
  Cytokines are small
  proteins that regulate
  immune responses.
  Researchers are
  investigating the use of
  cytokine therapies, such as
  interleukin-12 (IL-12) or
  interferon-gamma (IFN-
  gamma), to enhance the
  immune system's ability to
  clear Borrelia burgdorferi
  infections. These therapies
  aim to stimulate specific
  immune cells and promote

a more robust and targeted response against the bacteria.

- T-Cell Immunotherapy: T-cell immunotherapy involves using genetically engineered T-cells, a type of immune cell, to target and kill Borrelia-infected cells. This approach holds promise in directly attacking the bacteria and reducing the reservoir of persistent infection.

While immunotherapy for Lyme disease is still in its early stages, these approaches have shown encouraging results in preclinical studies and some early-phase clinical trials. However, further research is needed to determine their optimal dosing, safety profiles, and long-term efficacy.

2. Vaccines: Vaccines play a crucial role in preventing infectious diseases, and the development of an effective Lyme disease vaccine has been a long-standing goal in the field. Although a previous Lyme disease vaccine called LYMErix was available, it was withdrawn from the market due to concerns over rare side effects and low demand. However, researchers continue to explore new vaccine

candidates with improved
safety and efficacy profiles:

- Outer Surface Protein A
  (OspA) Vaccines: OspA is
  a surface protein on the
  Borrelia bacteria and is a
  target for vaccine
  development. LYMErix
  was an OspA-based
  vaccine. New OspA-based
  vaccine candidates are
  under investigation, with
  modifications to enhance
  their effectiveness and
  reduce potential side
  effects.

- Multivalent Vaccines:
  Multivalent vaccines aim to
  protect against multiple

strains or species of
Borrelia bacteria. Lyme
disease is caused by several
different Borrelia species,
and a multivalent vaccine
could provide broader
protection. Researchers are
working on developing
multivalent vaccines that
incorporate key surface
proteins from multiple
Borrelia strains.

- DNA Vaccines: DNA
  vaccines involve
  introducing genetic
  material encoding Borrelia
  proteins into the body to
  stimulate an immune
  response. This approach
  has shown promise in

preclinical studies, and early clinical trials are underway to evaluate the safety and efficacy of DNA vaccines for Lyme disease.

- Protein Subunit Vaccines: Protein subunit vaccines consist of purified proteins derived from the Borrelia bacteria. These vaccines focus on specific surface proteins or antigens that elicit a strong immune response without including whole bacteria. Protein subunit vaccines are being developed and evaluated for their potential in preventing Lyme disease.

The development of an effective and safe Lyme disease vaccine remains an active area of research. Vaccine candidates are undergoing rigorous preclinical and clinical testing to assess their immunogenicity, safety, and ability to confer long-lasting protection against Lyme disease.

It is important to note that both immunotherapy and vaccine development for Lyme disease face unique challenges. The complex nature of the Borrelia bacteria, the potential for persistent infection, and variations in disease presentation among individuals pose obstacles in developing universally effective treatments. However, advancements in immunotherapy and vaccine research offer hope for improved prevention, treatment, and management of Lyme disease.

immunotherapy and vaccines are emerging as cutting-edge research and potential treatments for Lyme disease. Immunotherapy approaches aim to boost the immune system's response against the Borrelia bacteria, while vaccine development focuses on providing protection against Lyme disease. These innovative strategies have shown promise in preclinical and early clinical studies, although further research is needed to refine their effectiveness, safety profiles, and long-term outcomes. Continued efforts in these areas will contribute to the development of new tools for preventing and treating Lyme disease, ultimately improving the lives of those affected by this complex and challenging condition.

Stem Cell Therapy

Stem cell therapy is an area of cutting-edge research that holds promise for various medical conditions, including Lyme disease. Stem cells are unique cells with the ability to differentiate into different types of cells in the body and possess regenerative properties. In the context of Lyme disease, stem cell therapy aims to harness the regenerative potential of stem cells to promote tissue repair, modulate the immune response, and alleviate symptoms. Here, we explore the current research and emerging treatments related to stem cell therapy for Lyme disease.

1. Mesenchymal Stem Cells (MSCs): Mesenchymal stem cells are a type of adult stem cell that can be isolated from various tissues, including bone marrow, adipose tissue (fat), and umbilical cord tissue. MSCs have been extensively studied for their

therapeutic potential in various conditions due to their immunomodulatory properties and ability to promote tissue regeneration.

In the context of Lyme disease, MSCs are being investigated for their potential to modulate the immune response, reduce inflammation, and enhance tissue repair. Preclinical studies have shown promising results, demonstrating that MSCs can suppress the activity of immune cells involved in Lyme disease pathogenesis and promote the regeneration of damaged tissues. However, clinical trials evaluating the safety and efficacy of MSCs for Lyme disease are still in their early stages.

2. Induced Pluripotent Stem Cells (iPSCs): Induced pluripotent stem cells are generated by reprogramming adult cells, such as skin cells, to revert to a pluripotent state. This means that they can differentiate into any cell type in the body. iPSCs have the potential to be used in regenerative medicine and can be directed to differentiate into specific cell types relevant to Lyme disease, such as neuronal cells or immune cells.

Researchers are exploring the possibility of using iPSCs to better understand the mechanisms of Lyme disease, study the effects of the Borrelia bacteria on different cell types, and develop personalized treatment approaches. However, iPSC-based therapies for Lyme disease are still in the early stages of development, and more research is needed to determine their safety, efficacy, and long-term effects.

3. Other Stem Cell Approaches: In addition to MSCs and iPSCs, other stem cell approaches are being explored for Lyme disease treatment. These

include hematopoietic stem cell transplantation (HSCT) and neural stem cell therapy.

- HSCT involves transplanting blood-forming stem cells to replenish the immune system. It is being investigated as a potential treatment for severe or persistent cases of Lyme disease where the immune system is compromised or ineffective in clearing the infection.

- Neural stem cell therapy focuses on utilizing stem cells that can differentiate into neuronal cells. This approach aims to repair nerve damage and alleviate symptoms associated with Lyme disease-related neurologic complications.

Research in stem cell therapy for Lyme disease is still in its early stages, and many questions remain unanswered. Safety, long-term effects, optimal dosing, and patient selection criteria are among the factors that need to be thoroughly studied in well-designed clinical trials. Close collaboration between scientists, clinicians, and regulatory bodies is crucial to ensure the ethical and responsible development of stem cell therapies for Lyme disease.

Other Promising Developments

In addition to the specific areas mentioned above, several other promising developments are shaping the landscape of Lyme disease research and emerging treatments. These developments include:

1. Nanotechnology: Nanotechnology involves the manipulation of materials at the nanoscale level. Researchers are exploring the use of nanotechnology in Lyme disease diagnosis and

treatment. This includes the development of nanosensors for more sensitive and specific detection of Borrelia bacteria and the use of nanomaterials for targeted delivery of therapeutic agents to infected tissues.

2. Gene Editing Technologies: Gene editing technologies, such as CRISPR-Cas9, hold potential for precise manipulation of the Borrelia genome. Researchers are investigating the use of these technologies to disrupt essential genes in the bacteria, rendering them

unable to cause disease or increasing their susceptibility to antibiotics.

3. Artificial Intelligence (AI): AI and machine learning algorithms have the potential to enhance Lyme disease diagnosis, prediction of disease outcomes, and treatment optimization. AI models can analyze complex datasets, identify patterns, and assist clinicians in making more accurate decisions.

4. Novel Antibiotic Therapies: Researchers are exploring alternative antibiotic

treatments for Lyme disease, including the repurposing of existing drugs and the development of new compounds. These approaches aim to overcome antibiotic resistance, target persistent forms of the bacteria, and improve treatment outcomes.

5. Host-Directed Therapies: Host-directed therapies focus on modulating the host's immune response to effectively control the infection. Researchers are investigating various approaches, such as immune stimulants,

immunomodulatory agents, and host-directed antimicrobial therapies, to bolster the immune system's ability to combat the Borrelia bacteria.

It is important to note that while these developments hold promise, they are still in the research and early experimental stages. Further investigations, preclinical studies, and well-designed clinical trials are necessary to establish their safety, efficacy, and optimal use in the context of Lyme disease.

stem cell therapy, along with other promising developments, is a rapidly evolving field in Lyme disease research and emerging treatments. Stem cells, such as MSCs and iPSCs, show potential for modulating the immune response, promoting tissue repair, and improving outcomes in Lyme disease. However, more research is needed to understand their mechanisms of action, optimize treatment protocols, and ensure their safety and long-term effectiveness. Other advancements, including nanotechnology, gene editing technologies, AI, novel antibiotic therapies, and host-directed therapies, are also reshaping the landscape of Lyme disease research. Continued scientific exploration and collaboration are essential to translate these cutting-edge research findings into safe, effective, and accessible treatments for individuals affected by Lyme disease.

CHAPTER 3

Preventing Lyme Disease

Tick Bite Prevention

Preventing tick bites is crucial for reducing the risk of Lyme disease. Ticks are most commonly found in wooded or grassy areas, so taking preventive measures when spending time outdoors can significantly lower the chances of being bitten. Here are some strategies for tick bite prevention:

1. Wear Protective Clothing: When venturing into tick-

prone areas, wear long sleeves, long pants, and closed-toe shoes. Tuck your pants into your socks or boots to prevent ticks from crawling up your legs. Choose light-colored clothing to make it easier to spot ticks.

2. Use Tick Repellents: Apply an EPA-registered tick repellent to exposed skin and clothing. Look for repellents that contain DEET, picaridin, or permethrin. Follow the instructions carefully when applying repellents, especially on children.

3. Perform Tick Checks: After spending time outdoors, thoroughly check your body and clothing for ticks. Pay close attention to areas such as the scalp, behind the ears, under the arms, around the waistline, and between the legs. Promptly remove any ticks you find.

4. Create Tick-Safe Landscapes: Make your yard less attractive to ticks by keeping the grass mowed short, removing leaf litter and brush, and creating a barrier between wooded areas and recreational spaces using gravel or wood chips.

5. Use Tick Control Products:
Consider treating your
outdoor clothing and gear
with permethrin, a tick-
killing insecticide. You can
also treat your yard with
acaricides, which target
ticks specifically.

CHAPTER 4

Protecting Your Living Environment

Ticks can enter your living space through various means, so taking steps to protect your environment can help prevent Lyme disease. Here are some measures to safeguard your living environment:

1. Keep Indoor Areas Clean: Regularly clean your living spaces, vacuum carpets, and remove clutter. Ticks can hide in cracks, crevices, and fabrics, so thorough

cleaning reduces their
hiding spots.

2. Create Tick Barriers: Apply
   a tick control product, such
   as diatomaceous earth or
   botanical pesticides, in
   areas where ticks may enter
   your home, such as near
   doors, windows, and crawl
   spaces. This can help deter
   ticks from entering your
   living space.

3. Pet Protection: Ticks can
   latch onto pets and be
   brought inside, increasing
   the risk of exposure to ticks
   for you and your family.
   Use tick prevention

products on your pets, such as tick collars or spot-on treatments. Regularly check your pets for ticks and promptly remove any you find.

4. Secure Outdoor Trash: Ticks are attracted to food sources, including discarded food scraps. Make sure your outdoor trash cans have tight-fitting lids to prevent animals that may carry ticks from accessing them.

5. Seal Entry Points: Seal any gaps, cracks, or openings in your home's exterior to prevent ticks from entering.

Pay attention to areas
where utility pipes, cables,
or wires enter the building.

CHAPTER 5

Recognizing Early Symptoms

Early recognition of Lyme disease symptoms is crucial for timely diagnosis and treatment. The hallmark sign of Lyme disease is the characteristic rash called erythema migrans (EM). However, not all individuals develop this rash, so it's important to be aware of other early symptoms, which can include:

1. Flu-like Symptoms: Fever, fatigue, chills, headache,

muscle and joint aches, and swollen lymph nodes are common flu-like symptoms that can occur in the early stages of Lyme disease.

2. Erythema Migrans (EM) Rash: This rash typically appears within 3 to 30 days after a tick bite and expands gradually. It often resembles a bull's-eye, with a central clearing surrounded by a red outer ring. However, the rash can vary in appearance and may not always have a distinctive pattern.

3. Other Skin Manifestations: In some cases, individuals

may develop multiple EM rashes or rashes that differ from the classic bull's-eye pattern. These rashes can occur on different parts of the body.

4. Neurological Symptoms: In rare cases, Lyme disease can cause neurological symptoms, such as meningitis, facial paralysis (Bell's palsy), and numbness or weakness in the limbs.

If you experience any of these symptoms, especially after a known tick bite or potential exposure to ticks, it is important to seek medical attention. Early diagnosis and treatment with appropriate antibiotics can effectively eliminate the infection and prevent the progression of Lyme disease.

By implementing tick bite prevention strategies, protecting your living environment, and being vigilant about early symptoms, you can significantly reduce the risk of Lyme disease and ensure timely medical intervention if needed.

CHAPTER 6

Living Well with Lyme Disease

Managing Symptoms and Flare-ups

Living with Lyme disease often involves managing symptoms and addressing occasional flare-ups. While treatment approaches may vary depending on individual circumstances, here are some strategies to help manage symptoms and navigate flare-ups:

1. Medication Management: Work closely with your

healthcare provider to develop a personalized medication regimen. This may include antibiotics to target the infection, pain relievers for symptom management, and other medications to address specific symptoms or complications.

2. Symptom Tracking: Keep a symptom journal to monitor your symptoms, their severity, and potential triggers. This can help you identify patterns and make informed decisions regarding lifestyle adjustments, treatment

modifications, or seeking medical advice.

3. Lifestyle Modifications: Adopting a healthy lifestyle can support symptom management and overall well-being. This includes getting regular exercise (at a level suitable for your condition), eating a balanced diet, prioritizing adequate sleep, and managing stress through relaxation techniques, such as meditation or yoga.

4. Pain Management Techniques: Explore various pain management strategies, such as heat or

cold therapy, physical therapy, acupuncture, or massage. Additionally, practicing stress reduction techniques, such as deep breathing exercises or mindfulness, can help alleviate pain and promote relaxation.

5. Recognize and Respect Your Limits: Understand your energy levels and limitations, and pace yourself accordingly. Pushing beyond your limits can potentially exacerbate symptoms or trigger flare-ups. Listen to your body and practice self-care by resting when needed.

Building Resilience and Self-Care Strategies

Living with Lyme disease can be physically and emotionally challenging. Building resilience and adopting self-care strategies can empower you to navigate the ups and downs of your condition. Consider the following approaches:

1. Emotional Well-being: Acknowledge and validate your emotions surrounding Lyme disease. Seek support from mental health professionals, join support groups, or engage in therapy to help manage

anxiety, depression, or other emotional challenges.

2. Stress Management: Develop effective stress management techniques, such as practicing relaxation exercises, engaging in hobbies or activities that bring joy, spending time in nature, or pursuing creative outlets. Finding healthy ways to manage stress can positively impact your overall well-being.

3. Mind-Body Practices: Explore mind-body practices, such as meditation, deep breathing

exercises, or guided
imagery, to promote
relaxation, reduce stress,
and improve emotional
well-being. These practices
can also help alleviate
symptoms and enhance
resilience.

4. Sleep Hygiene: Prioritize
   quality sleep by
   establishing a consistent
   sleep routine, creating a
   comfortable sleep
   environment, and practicing
   relaxation techniques
   before bedtime. Good sleep
   hygiene can contribute to
   overall health and well-
   being.

5. Prioritize Self-Care: Make self-care a priority by engaging in activities that bring you joy, practicing self-compassion, and setting boundaries. This may include activities like reading, spending time with loved ones, pursuing hobbies, or engaging in gentle exercises that align with your energy levels.

Nurturing Relationships and Support Networks

Nurturing relationships and building a support network can be invaluable when living with Lyme disease. Here are some ways to foster connections and seek support:

1. Educate Loved Ones: Help your family, friends, and loved ones understand Lyme disease by providing them with educational resources or encouraging them to attend support groups or educational sessions. This can foster empathy, support, and understanding.

2. Seek Support: Connect with others who have Lyme disease through local support groups, online communities, or social media platforms. Sharing

experiences, exchanging information, and receiving support from individuals who understand your journey can be empowering and comforting.

3. Communicate Your Needs: Clearly communicate your needs, limitations, and boundaries to your support network. This can help them provide appropriate support and adjust expectations accordingly.

4. Engage in Open Dialogue: Maintain open and honest communication with your healthcare providers, expressing any concerns or

questions you may have. Establishing a collaborative relationship with your healthcare team can enhance your understanding of treatment options and improve your overall care.

5. Professional Support: Consider seeking the assistance of a therapist, counselor, or Lyme-literate healthcare provider who specializes in Lyme disease. These professionals can provide guidance, support, and specific strategies for navigating the challenges of living with Lyme disease.

Remember that living well with Lyme disease is a journey unique to each individual. It's essential to tailor these strategies to your specific needs, seek professional guidance when necessary, and embrace a holistic approach to self-care, resilience-building, and nurturing relationships.

9 798399 917849